WELLNESS UNVEILED

WELLNESS UNVEILED

JUDE HAWTHORNE

CONTENTS

CHAPTER 1

Introduction to Wellness and Its Importance

"Wednesday's Child is full of woe" is a chant we all grew up with. Then research in the late 1980s showed that children who were labeled as "ticking time bombs" would become depressed, give up on life, drink, use drugs, then commit suicide. It was discovered that an early symptom of this outcome was apathy; it became clear that unless an individual cared about self, there was little reason for going on. Psychologists concluded that it was in the individual's self-interest to care for and about self. They now call this "self-development," the concept of wellness. As educators, we see wellness as something that must be maintained to establish balance in human beings. Wellness is rooted in the person's wisdom and his wants. By addressing an individual and his wants, it becomes easier to set goals for self-actualization. The human spirit becomes involved in the process.

The complex of standard health models includes the anatomical, physiological, psychological, and social dimensions of health, while the wellness models that have been looked at include: (1) the psychodynamic model of the physical thinker, (2) an enthusiastic call to increased spirituality as a dimension of full personal satisfaction, and

(3) the physical, social, and spiritual model. Clearly, defining wellness is problematic and it is easy to become lost in the maze of philosophical differences. Despite the disagreements concerning wellness' roots, wellness is a concept that has gained increased attention in the language of health around the world. People and healthcare professionals are beginning to label efforts that prevent the acquisition of diseases as "wellness" activities.

Defining Wellness and Its Components

A. DC defines wellness as the freedom not only from disease and discomfort, but the conditions that cause such disease and discomfort. B. In essence, the dialogue engaged in with the individual experiencing the disease or discomfort includes information about why illness occurs and the steps the individual can take to prevent illness and increase the likelihood of greater health. C. The heart of the DC's wellness care role is patient education. D. The DC supports the individual in each chosen or created dimension of their life. E. These dimensions of wellness or good health are: The ability of the body to handle all physical activities. The ability to carry out daily tasks with vigor and alertness, without undue fatigue, and with ample energy to enjoy leisure time pursuits and to meet unforeseen emergencies. The ability to get along with others, to establish mutual relationships, and to influence others in a positive way. This includes leadership and teamwork. The capacity to identify one's own feelings and the capability of coping with them and with emotional challenges and stress. The achievement of personal fulfillment in work and play which is in harmony with one's value system, and which is beneficial to one's individual and collective community.

In practice, the DCs at Logan uphold these dimensions of wellness through our commitment to providing a superior education for our students, treating patients in the University Health Centers, and maintaining our own health-care practices throughout our lives. G. While recognizing that the partnership between the patient and the practitioner is of the utmost importance, the Faculty Wellness Committee has established the following program recommendations as supportive activities and guidelines for leading a personally effective, socially responsible life. H. The Doctor of Chiropractic degree is designed not only to permit the graduate to apply, but understand and promote the dimensions of wellness. The program develops knowledge and understanding of leadership and teamwork so the chiropractor can participate in multidisciplinary referral networks, and to encourage students to become personally effective, socially responsible, and effective members of society. I. Guidelines for leading a personally effective, socially responsible life. The DC has established the independence in daily living to help ensure a healthy planet. J. As leaders, Logan graduates are committed to living in an ethical manner and have the knowledge and integrity to balance personal and professional life. K. To assist in the development of each of these components, the Doctor of Chiropractic Program teaches and encourages participation in wellness services that are based upon a comprehensive view, rather than narrowly focused in one area. The faculty and staff of Logan are committed to upholding each of these wellness components as exemplified by the activities of the departmental and university committees.

The Significance of Wellness in Modern Society

The word 'wellness' in contemporary society has been influenced by various forces including personal health concerns, business economics, and the pressures of urbanization. Over time, the concept of wellness has grown to a point where it is of significance to all modern societies. Modern medicine's ability to deal successfully with major health issues has seen a shift in public perception as to what constitutes a 'healthy society'. In addition, urbanization and its associated lifestyle challenges have underlined the fact that there is much more to wellness than the absence of sickness. Clearly defined prerequisites for internationally accepted wellness principles and practices are essential for benchmarking global wellness standards that promote the highest achievable competencies, skills, and knowledge necessary to maintain and enhance physical well-being, personal achievement, sense of life direction, and healthy condition of the person.

Wellness has evolved as a major theme in society despite there being no available, widely disseminated, and agreed definition. There is no stopping the wellness phenomenon as the quest for the standard of human potential grows. Wellness or health awareness is not only an essential component of modern society but has grown to be one of the largest industries in response to health concerns. These concerns have led to the creation of countless wellness fads, directly linked to increases in consumerism and the willingness of the public to accept a variety of promises that wellness solutions bring. There are few wholly 'well' people in society. These are few and far between, mostly present as buffs who participate in a variety of activities displaying a perfection often unobtainable by the person on the street.

CHAPTER 2

Historical Perspectives on Wellness

The origins of the wellness concept are rooted in ancient history. The symbols of longevity and well-being, which have evolved from early pictographic to modern alphabetic forms, are expressed to a large extent in language and are also found in printed and online texts as well as in logos, signs, symbols, and other forms of communication about well-being. While some of these artifacts and representations are well known and widely recognized, many are artifacts of forgotten origins and lost meanings. Interdisciplinary research on wellness makes it possible to unravel the meanings and reveal the healing powers in these artifacts and words, which can be either ancient or modern expressions of the health dialogue. Such studies in wellness philology provide the foundation for a comprehensive dialogue on health and well-being knowledge that encompasses a broad array of human activities, including but not limited to oral, hypnosis, physical, energetic, intuitive, and spiritual healing.

Early intervention and health diagnostic strategies are proposed based on matching individual ontological attributes with wellness modalities. The practical approaches to wellness interventions and wellness assessment include SoulIntensity© assessment, physical agility evaluations, movement assessments, and beyond. These and other wellness measurement modalities require further validation and demonstration before they are considered ready for field use. Ultimately, multiple modalities provide assessments of ontological strengths, weaknesses, opportunities, and threats using various combinations and permutations of the descriptors and their attributions. Based on these ontological assessments, personalized wellness programs are to be developed and offered.

Ancient Practices and Beliefs

The ideas underpinning wellness are not new. Rather, they draw on ancient practices and beliefs that stretch back to at least 3000 BC. Belief systems in various cultures believe that 'correct' physical and mental forces are essential for good health. Chinese health promotion emphasizes getting the flow of energy within the body right, Taoists seek to unite their inner spirit with the spirit of the whole, and health promoting Native American Indians also strive for a harmonious link with nature. Likewise, Ayurvedic medicine emphasizes how to care for the body in such a way as to live in harmony not only with oneself but with all living things. Hence, in ancient India, serious thought was given to social and spiritual dimensions. To be fully healthy the liver must function perfectly, explained Plato. Thoughts such as these laid the foundation for the wellness belief system.

Wellness is not new but does incorporate other steps disallowed in individual belief systems, particularly with respect to the general levels of knowledge and sophistication brought about by education and science. Extending wellness beliefs to the mainstream through the health system formalizes and legitimizes that which many already seek. The seven components of wellness that Ddwl described in 1976 still sound quite appropriate, covering the social, intellectual, spiritual, and physical dimensions. Now there are others and so diverse is the work that Dr Mullings remarked how remarkable it is that there is general acceptance of wellness as a viable state of being in western societies.

Evolution of Wellness Concepts

Health is recognized as one of the renewable resources of any nation. Over time, the concept of health has evolved. It has been recognized that health is a multidimensional concept. The idea that wellness is multidimensional is not new. Through the ages, ancient philosophical systems such as Indian and Chinese have made references to the concept of wellness as a state of being.

Susruta, an Indian philosopher who lived in the 6th century BC, classified mental health conditions such as Unmada. He presented 3 types: possession by evil spirits, alterations of personality, and the epileptic syndrome which appears to the community in accordance with modern symptoms. Also, two other categories of disturbance such as Parinamashana (Climacteric) and Akasmathsanya (Posttraumatic Stress Disorder) and preventive aspects of mental illness were described earlier.

The concept of mental health has been understood in different ways in different times and societies throughout history, and its practical aspects have been expressed in an infinite number of customs, rituals, exorcisms, and therapies. When examining the history of psychiatric nursing, we find the fundamental influence of the health-disease paradigm that characterizes the culture of a certain period. It was Freud and his psychoanalysis that fundamentally modified the perspective of man to explain behaviors, identifying human beings as carriers of the instincts, functioning in a way that is later minimized, transforming individuals into neurotics and psychotic patients.

CHAPTER 3

Physical Wellness

The most crucial and directly health-related dimension of wellness is physical wellness. It refers to keeping a healthy body and seeking healthy lifestyle choices. This sentiment is echoed by Anastasia Rights and Liz Stevens, who remarked that "positive physical health contributes to one's overall well-being." As already argued in the opening chapter of this book, the prominence of the physical dimension to wellness comes from the considerable research base that highlights the significant relationship between physical health and psychological well-being. Taking short breaks to walk around outdoor gardens or courtyards can help to release stress arising from work pressure or anything else. Parks and gardens also provide a setting for exercise (e.g., walking, badminton, aerobics, and stretching) and maintaining a healthy lifestyle. Being uncomfortable with obesity is not solely because obesity is not aesthetically pleasing; it is because obesity is a clear indication of ill health. It is well-documented that obesity is a risk factor for various health problems. It is clearly an impediment to living life to the fullest.

Nutrition and Diet

The term "wellness" has been in greater evidence today in the literature, popular press, and media venues than in the past and is generally used in reference to human health and well-being. Wellness is an exciting and challenging field that could be developed as a philosophy, belief, or as a science. For example, a philosophy of wellness would include value judgments and arguments about what human beings ought to do in order to be well, while a scientific approach would seek to assess the degree of human well-being and the responsibility that individuals, professions, corporations, and the state would have in securing the well-being. In either approach, wellness could be considered as a necessary aspect of ethical reflection. As a philosophy, wellness is a good to be sought, especially if, as some suggest, wellness is an end-in-itself.

Wellness is important for managers who recognize pressures of time and complexity in the workplace and for the consultants responsible for organizational doings. In many banks and in other service-oriented industries, professionals are under increased pressure to perform and to meet an ongoing series of organizational pressures. Since wellness seems to involve some sort of caring, in a corporate context, wellness implies a level of attention to the multi-dimensional satisfaction of material and personal needs which have not hitherto been a primary interest of many corporations. Notwithstanding whether wellness should properly be seen as a field of applied ethics, the private and professional gains for any individual (or for any organization) committed to wellness are probably unambiguous. Despite grassroots interest in the concept, major corporate leaders, as a rule, have been slow to embrace wellness as a critical component of their corporate strategies. Yet, some, with high stature and respect, such as the banking leader, Warren Buffet, have embraced it. They have seen that their long-term success is dependent on the wellness of their employees.

Exercise and Physical Activity

Exercise includes physical movement and motion that work to affect physical exertion. Physical activity involves any bodily movement performed by skeletal muscles and results in the utilization of energy. It increases the caloric demand over resting energy expenditures and is essential in maintaining overall economy and preventing calorie storage as fat. Typical physical activities include mild office activities, heavy outdoor activities, and intense schooling. Anyone who does not engage in regular physical activity is not practicing proper exercise.

Physical exercise is a personally structured regimen consisting of physical training, durations, and maintenance. Fitness activities are carried out through organized and functional-class activities, regular and personalized routines, and adjusted recovery and relaxation. In basic hospital treatment, concentrated exercise is crucial for individuals who need to improve their fitness levels. For those who are not taking strong medications and are in the process of recovering strength, incorporating physical exercises into their daily lives is important.

This requires a reassessment of activity and sitting for individuals or populations, taking into account their weaknesses, strengths, obstacles, and limitations. This level of work involves the use of energy or effort when discussing the exercise of body systems, enhancing technical properties, and improving our skills to generate more energy and flexibility. Exercises can be included in a health-related activity framework, structured by a profession or wellness team or leadership group, or managed by the individual themselves, to meet specific physical, social, medical, and other exercise requirements.

Sleep and Rest

Although sleep is now coming to the forefront and being recognized as the most important aspect of wellness in our lives, we must remember that the body goes into a rest state when this is done properly. This rest allows the body to rehydrate and prepare to wake up and start anew. The hours we sleep do not predict the quality of rest, and the fact that we spiral into light sleep after 4 hours and cycle every 2 hours per sleep night becomes a part of your picture, which ensures the mind receives all it needs to prepare and recuperate to function for the following day and store all we have learned into long-term memory.

This is the only time the body gets a chance to repair any damage done during the day, and the rest system allows the body to rest, repair, and get ready for the next dawn. Without sleep, serious mental and physical health problems can occur. If wellness embraces all aspects of your life, then this base wellness pattern must be proper sleep and proper rest. Unfortunately, 45% of adults state that lack of sleep makes it difficult to concentrate at work or home. When I reflect on my children, it is easy to see how the pattern always repeats itself. I had forgotten those times.

CHAPTER 4

Mental and Emotional Wellness

In medicine, mental and emotional wellness hinge predominantly around the effects and aspects of wellness that determine the cognitive experience one has of the world and how one handles that world from a feelings standpoint - the fundamental unit of cognition being a thought. Since our discussions will relate mostly to person, we will separate this into the two foundational but not separate aspects of mental and emotional wellness. In reality, the two aspects are an integrated aspect which we, human beings, call person. Mental wellness encompasses everything to do with the way in which we think and the way we use our cognitive faculties, in other words the fruit of our evolutionary process that can require this. Emotional wellness concerns various parallel aspects of wellness that have to do with the quality and efficacy of our physical well-being, integration, and mental well-being, but the component aspect of wellness should not be greatly overshadowed by it as has been so common in the philosophical history of the human race.

Emotional wellness has four key aspects, all in essence required for self-awareness, awareness of others, of the world in which we live, and of the truth that underpins it. First, those components, wellness and mental health, have to be present to some extent. Any abnormal affective response could signal a competition between wellness, mental health, and one's way of experiencing the world. Second, also comprising the ability to assess and confront the outside world and so skilled action, emotion in a healthy state also relies on mental well-being. Finally, emotion has, to some extent, to depend on an awareness of reality and a philosophical understanding to make it clear that an afterlife in a personal myth created by our ancestors is not always real.

Stress Management

The American Institute of Stress refers to stress as the "being allergic to life" syndrome. Stress is all around us, at home, at work, every time we are exposed to a tune change in our affairs. And we do need this change: music, for instance, to be and remain entertaining, appealing, fresh, does depend on tune changes. However, as our audio systems can be damaged by and unhappy with the sudden and excessive variation between the same day-to-day exposure to silence and a full-volume rock concert, we can harm our mental and physical wellness by "living" on a stress-embraced life. Therefore, we must learn to soften this tune change because the hard truth is that, no matter the theory and dreams, life implies duty and duty implies stress. The mindful human is aware of this definitional postulate of reality and lives accordingly, drawing the life balance between cinema and caring, soft music.

The Coimbra Ayurveda Study provides us with essential tools we need to succeed in stress redemption - exploring the universe within (our own specific inner biochemistry which includes our mental and behavioral specifics, and is accountable by life choices and influences) and looking outward to Earth's ecosystem to better attend and manage life duties. Emotional intelligence (frequent self-assaults through kindness, empathy and compassion, among others), communion (the "old girl from Coimbra", which says "there is not me without the others and there are not the others without me"), and introspective reflection (relatively frequent sun baths of uniqueness) orbit around stress management in the wellness galaxy because none of them accomplishes their main tasks out of the better aura stress management provides. And this stimulus extends to the whole wide spectrum of living. The area of Suggestive Medicine shows this to us with an exception - the command action volunteer. However, always avoid excessive habitual impulsiveness situations that, we should remind you, are quite capable of swarming life rocks between five-day and five-day "island waits".

Mental Health Awareness and Stigma

In addition to promoting candid dialogue on mental health as a wellness element, the Health Dialogue also emphasized the issue of stigma. Best Health Canada research indicates that despite the majority of Canadian employees thinking mental health is important and only 23% opposing the mental health awareness coverage, it is estimated that only one third of employees would feel comfortable discussing a mental health problem in the workplace, and only 25% would talk to their manager. The Conference Board of Canada's survey revealed that one-fifth of all respondents could learn that a colleague had a serious illness or mental illness, be concerned that their future may be harmed, and avoid having lunch with them. The Canadian Social Research Council's survey - mental health in Canada found that 22% of individuals describe themselves as having "shyness, shame, guilt, or judgment" as mental health-related barriers, 18% have doubts about privacy, 16% fear prejudice and discrimination, and 9% are afraid that they will need to use legal or workplace "backlash" services.

This Health Dialogue project provides several key recommendations to reduce workplace mental health stigma. Conduct an orientation to develop the full support and support of the leadership. Openly encourage a dialogue on mental health awareness. Cover requirements, share personal stories, and/or volunteer to organize and promote various mental health-related activities. Empower employees to engage in mental health through education, training, and resources. It can merge these best practices into the organization's action proposals. Strive to establish a community culture that emphasizes that everyone's mental health is being supported and sees mental health support as an important and active part of the broader aspects of wellness. Promote the establishment of advisory groups that not only express the views and needs of intra-mental health and development but also help monitor the effectiveness of the mental health initiative. Best Health Canada research provides clear suggestions and tools to implement these recommendations through Mental Health at Work. The management organization can further recognize the significance of awareness and stigma reduction by seeking Mental Health at Work Certification.

CHAPTER 5

Social Wellness

The ability of individuals to interact effectively with others and to develop satisfying and supportive relationships is a fundamental aspect of wellness. Social wellness is of particular importance as modern institutions place individuals in stressful and ambiguous environments where supportive relationships are essential to coping with the surrounding ambiguity and pressures. Family and other vital relationships often suffer as a result of the significant contribution to be made within an organization or a profession. Many, however, find it increasingly difficult to fulfill the demands both of their work and their family and personal lives.

The technological society also places individuals in a world where communications often become superficial and non-existent, and surfaces obscure personal ties. The phenomenon of the commuter suburbs, for example, is often cited as an indicator of the degree to which community life has declined. In the electronic age, human and institutional relationships have become easier to form, but the ease of forming such relationships has resulted in many that are not deeply rooted and therefore easily broken. People can travel anywhere and communicate with anyone in the world. But as they exercise their opportunities for free movement and unrestricted communication, people become more isolated, lonelier, and less self-sufficient in their daily lives. It may be that social wellness depends upon a personal capacity to connect local with global, personal with institutional, and to appropriately balance the public and private aspects of experience.

Importance of Relationships and Social Support

We demonstrated a considerable body of literature on the importance of relationships and social support to physical and mental health. Both the amount of contact and the perceived quality of relationships are important. Relationships impact health through their ability to relieve stress and depression, improve self-esteem, provide meaning and purpose in life, and encourage self-care and health maintenance. Positive social and emotional support is correlated with fast recovery from illness, less pain, and better general health. The sensations of anxiety, sadness, helplessness, and abandonment tend to improve and reduce pain. In conclusion, supportive relationships have a number of health benefits, and the social consequences of being ill or disabled are minimized for those patients with sustained social contact. We also listed several group programs that have been established in order to combat the impact of social isolation and loneliness.

All too often, however, the negative effects of social support for those individuals who enjoy good health and a vibrant social network are overlooked. Indeed, the benefits of being a confidant and good listener to one's circle of friends are beneficial to health in their own right. Alzheimer's patients are good examples: their primary and active relationship with the couple providing the most support for them is more likely to be longer, with greater experience of providing support, and many more hours of such support each month. Other successful interventions in the relationship include psychoeducation programs that have improved the capability of partners to provide competent care to their loved ones with Alzheimer's symptoms. This could be attributed to the ability of the couple to cope with stress and pressure, which in effect strengthens their relationship and reduces the physical complaints of the Alzheimer's patient. Overall, these findings indicate that health is a key factor in determining relationship outcomes.

Community Engagement and Well-Being

We describe the community engagement of six CBPR research projects aimed at increasing the individual well-being of community-dwelling older adults. Community members, irrespective of age, play a critical role in the lives of older adults. As part of the community, they offer insight into area resources and support and have access to informal and formal networks that can provide assistance. Even though several researchers have recognized the importance that seniors place on community involvement, to our knowledge, no systematic study has examined the relationship between the impact of community barriers and enrolled older subjects in CBPR interventions. We describe the community engagement of six CBPR research projects aimed at increasing the individual well-being of community-dwelling older adults. Additionally, we describe the sampling protocols, study design, and characteristics of the organizations, their patrons, staff, and senior participants.

As of now, we are unaware of systematic research that has addressed either of these questions, leaving an important gap in our knowledge of reciprocity: to what extent do community members who participate in our communities both benefit from and contribute to our communities, and how might the strength of that dynamic contribute to the premiere health, social and personal outcomes that many cities seek to achieve. We also describe the characteristics of the projects, staff, and community engagement strategies.

Then we evaluate intra- and interorganizational relationships and draw implications for wellness and expertise networks. Despite these benefits that are available from the attendance to and participation in existing and potential programs, up to 60% of the older population is hesitant to engage in many activities. This is troubling because the lack of social engagement can considerably limit an older person's quality of life.

CHAPTER 6

Environmental Wellness

Environmental wellness recognizes the interrelatedness of humans, nature, and the universe. It informs us of the following two points: the interactions of antibody and environmental forces, and the idea of environmental liability. The quality of air, water, and land, as well as the physical wellbeing of animals and plants, is an integral component of environmental wellness. Occupying comforting, exciting communities, and contributing to others who live in them as well as to the decline of the world's atmosphere are all examples of good environmental attributes. You will affirm the environment of the earth.

Particular air controls, cool water sources, decent homes, social communities, and secure streets are some examples of factors that can improve the atmosphere in which our citizens live. A healthy living environment for people is a healthy body. When we learn more about causes of environmental impairment, we will become aware that each creature is responsible for the welfare of our environment, which leads to environmental sensitivity.

Impact of Environment on Health and Well-Being
Good environmental quality and well-being are closely interlinked. It ensures minimal risks of infectious and non-infectious

diseases and fosters healthy and sustainable ecosystems through its links to human health, economy, and society. In developing regions, it will play a crucial part, with challenges due to rapid industrial growth and urbanization, and the reliance on more traditional and smaller scale sources, often located in regions with poor environmental management. There are numerous examples in history where improvements to the infrastructure and management have led to rises in life expectancy, growth in economic activity, and improvements within local society. These encompass fresh air ventilation during the London Plague, clean water supplies to prevent diseases, the sewage system correlation to the longevity of the Paris water project, and the success of the vaccination of children's programs globally.

An additional driver for addressing environmental health is the current popularity of the value under the sustainable development agenda. Moving from a business as usual practice of their prevailing approach to a sustainable and interconnected approach to both environmental and social dimensions creates additional responsibilities for discovering, not only the fields in the environmental health area that may have contributory paybacks, but also the proactive manner of discovering and addressing potential threats. This will also have gain add-on influences as many of the issues debated within the environmental sector, for example pollution of air and water, are also those that the wider society at a global, national, community or individual level are concerned about or directly affected by. Furthermore, a successful conclusion of the different international protocols that champion this is an outstanding opportunity to ensure maintaining a healthy and appropriate environment for all, especially those who are more vulnerable.

The traditionally comprehensive areas for environmental health are also the more recognized by society. The proactive agenda includes those which are often considered to be discrete by looking at them interactively, and also disregards topical issues, where environmental health is not frequently perceived to have a role at all. As such, the relevance of environmental health on human health and government and policy decisions appears to be frequently underestimated. For example, at a global level the joint WHO/GEF health and environment linkage initiative shows that only 88 of the over hundred and ninety Nation health plans identified had identifying linking health and environment. The study also aimed that only a number of the reviews recognized the part played by the global ecosystem which maintained the well-being of the human population. Reported cases of vector-borne infections frequently ignore the local environment and only pay attention to the clinical management of the patient. Another example is the lack of a more recent environmental health risk register, such as the US Department of Health and Human Services', whose responsibility is to approve experts to review and concur with hasty opinions if an environmental event occurred. Being involved in preventing and minimizing the effect of public health emergencies due to Ebola, Middle East respiratory disease, and avian influenza, made it essential to also have the necessary information to address the public health consequences. Not only was the environmental health voice not there, but society at large, including policymakers at the European Union and member state levels, did not regard it relevant to have input on environmental health. Succinctly, reinforcing the part of environmental health in health policies would partly reflect the understanding of the value of maintaining a healthy environment for societies, economies, and world health organizations.

Sustainable Living Practices

Every day, in ways we don't even realize, we impact the environment. The impact is mostly negative. We pollute the air, soil, and water. We compromise the health and lives of animals. And in consuming nonrenewable resources, we may leave the future with fewer resources than the present. Moreover, as a result of current consumption patterns, the people of the more developed nations are taking a larger share of the world's resources, leaving minimal above-subsistence levels for most of the Third World population. Many individuals are increasingly desiring to live in ways that minimize the damage done to the ecosystems. By taking another look at how we use and abuse the world's lands, waters, plant resources, and animal resources, we can start living and consuming sustainably. We can strive to live within the boundaries of the biosphere's ability to provide the resources we need and to absorb our wastes.

The ways we affect the environment can generally be classified into six categories. This project will explore the obvious and perhaps not-so-obvious ways we impact the environment and introduce some creative ideas for minimizing the impacts. Recognizing that variations and exceptions may apply, we will focus on the overall contribution an individual can make in each area. The six primary impacts of lifestyle on the environment are energy consumption, water demands, land use, resource consumption, pollutants output, and waste output.

CHAPTER 7

Spiritual Wellness

For centuries, scientists have been interested in studying the human spirit. Spiritual wellness involves the search for significant meaning and purpose in human existence, which may involve the development of a close relationship with a higher power, a belief in practices or values that support the idea that life cannot be separated from itself, or the explanation of phenomena individuals transcendence of themselves, in community or in the environment can contribute to wellness. Spiritual activities can include reading spiritual books or literature, meditating, praying, going to church, looking at art or creating art, doing yoga, spending time sunbathing and outdoors, performing service, spending time exalting something as beautiful, and a variety of other activities. When personal beliefs are acquired and become a unity with behavior, a flow of some sort arises. Whether spiritual wellness is consistently high or low as a result of spiritual belief, it is the search for meaning and satisfaction in human life that contributes to health, happiness, and optimal bearing out in life.

Faith and sacrifice are important to spiritual wellness. It builds happiness and peace of mind to have a solid faith that triggers certain lifestyle sequences, which by themselves increase mental, physical, and spiritual health and reduce the fear of COVID-19. Faith unites with total being and propels human beings. Those who value their spiritual tradition and spiritual adult reason experience meaningful situations and activities in life, and associate to all to live a life intended to cultivate exclusive relationships with the whole cosmos, themselves, society, and the superordinary, whether the supreme being is defined as divine. Truly, the guidelines of living – religious beliefs and spirituality – may link revolutionary science and spiritual liberation to assert a well-balanced mental, physical, and spiritual health. The evolution of an exclusive perspective warrants spiritual wellness, which is bounded in one's belief or veneration and is applied in the form of self-discipline and supplication. Whether the belief is to choose family responsibility, voluntary service, one's association with a supreme being, time in solitude and meditation, or the pursuit of understanding gospel power, accountability, and opulence elements, spiritual mindfulness should be observed in a BPS wellness initiative.

Exploring Belief Systems and Values

Within any given ethnic or cultural group, and in fact within any given society or group, its members share a system of shared values - a "map" of the world, which sometimes becomes so intrinsic that their actions are dictated by such beliefs. In discussing their health concerns, their accounts of their diseases, or indeed any health-related beliefs, we must see them in the total context of their value system. Unfortunately, the influence on morals and values on health, both positively in the encouraging of health, and negatively in the sense of being pathogenic, are virtually uncatalogued and unexplored. This is not overstating the case. Good health is generally considered in the modern world to be one of society's values, very much in the same way and with the same moral overtones as is honesty, industry, sobriety, loyalty, and all those personal qualities encapsulated in the emotionally-laden term "community virtues." Just as the "other" virtues bear messages, so too does health, and in the messages about illness which the "sick" bring to society.

The nature of such messages and the response are of considerable importance to doctors. The professional classes concerned with the sick and with making the sick well, or rather with advising on how the individual can become well - apart from the clergy, and today even the clergy are in retreat - are the principal focus of normative behaviors. Their concerns, the symptoms of illness and the search for its cure, all have an ethical, moral or normative message that affects every level of the community. The malingerer is the principal moral hazard of the provider of social service. On the other hand, the ill are entitled to the care of a physician as of right. Why? Because of entitlements defined by need, maintained by wealth, or dignity, because of their station in life, their status in society, because it's good business, for any, or perhaps all of these reasons. The morality play of the responsibilities, one to the other, is re-enacted again and again in boardrooms, general practitioner's consulting rooms, health departments, the world over. Banal perhaps, but illustrative of the way that intersecting belief systems unobtrusively shape the expectations of all concerned. These hidden beliefs, and the resultant behaviors, form the base of all dialogue about the illness or potential illness of a given individual, and are the crucible of the health dialogue in the community.

Mindfulness and Meditation

Mindfulness - the concept of being okay right now, happy right now - is extremely challenging and requires practice. The essence of mindfulness is to relax into the moment as it is, rather than spending so much time wanting something else or wanting what is not. Practices that help formalize becoming more mindful include deep breathing, meditation, and yoga. With practice, students usually find they are less restless and resistant to being in the moment, more focused, and better able to solve problems and express themselves. They are less anxious experiencing the daily chatter of their mental frontiers and more capable of entering a focused state of relaxed attention at any time they choose. Data suggest that a continuum of mindfulness skills lines up with a continuum of mental health, with mild to severe mental health issues impacting skills.

Increased resilience involves preparing the body and the mind to deal with the pressures of the learning process. Resilience includes learning to turn down the volume of angry, anxious thoughts, rather than following each negative feeling out to its extreme conclusion, improving the chance for calm, responsible behavior. Regular practices of strengthening the well-being include tai chi, meditation, deep breathing, and yoga. Any opportunity to practice or enhance resilience is important for students on the mental health continuum, but individuals on the left side of the bell curve often sustain high levels of focus, retention of information, and potentially greater benefit from specific strategies, including technology-supported strategies. Specialized techniques can calm the body and the nervous system while improving and reinforcing essential coping mechanisms.

CHAPTER 8

Occupational Wellness

Occupational wellness is the ability to achieve workplace satisfaction and fulfillment, take pride in what one does, and be recognized for contributions to the health dialogue. Research has shown that those who are able to integrate their passion and work have a lower risk of mortality, a slower rate of functional decline associated with aging, lower levels of depression, and retire later. Occupational wellness requires identifying what we are most passionate about and matching this with a suitable form of employment or recreation.

Work can become more than just a means to pay the bills. It can be a pathway to personal illumination, fulfillment, expansion, and happiness. To gain occupational wellness, one must enjoy work that is consistent with one's values, goals, lifestyle, and desired lifestyle. In the modern workplace, an individual's commitment to their occupation can add to personal satisfaction and success. The development of occupational wellness opens the organization to everyone's unique gifts, skills, and knowledge. This information provides self-aware team players who learn and contribute effectively in the changing world of work. A professionally occupational dimension combines the desire to live life to its fullest, with a built-in responsible sense of social consciousness. Health dialogue calls for mature therapists who are an advocate for wellness themselves. These individuals know the power of living life fully in the present. To fully enjoy this dimension of occupational wellness, one must obtain work satisfaction, attain an enriched professional and personal life, maintain a healthy balance between work and leisure time, create harmony in one's life employing a few strategies, and enjoy being part of the working environment.

Work-Life Balance

In its simplest form, work-life balance would seem to be the proportion and quality of time that we give to work compared with our out-of-work lives. There are, though, a number of ways in which the work-life balance can be distorted. Some of these are straightforward and do not happen very often - the short-term duty-week where one hardly sees home or curriculum night that takes over the world for a few days. These are regrettable instances of short-term pressure. However, chronic imbalances in work-life arrangements can encompass two separable strands - imbalances in individual lives and imbalances in working lives.

On the individual side, work-life imbalances are seen in the prevalence of fatigue, lowered levels of participation in family and community activities, and feelings of pressured confinement. Over on the working life side, imbalances are visible as loss of bonding with work tasks, loss of employee wellbeing (e.g., frustration, withdrawal, lowered morale), decreased efficiency at work, and a low fulfillment in work roles. Those with chronic imbalances are frequently doing work, whether paid or domestic, they do not want to do or they are doing them in a manner they do not like. Perspectives among practitioners and researchers are expanding from gender issues to review how work-life balance is different for groups experiencing the double disadvantage of poor health and low income.

Job Satisfaction and Fulfillment

From a wellness perspective, job satisfaction has been identified as the precondition to wellness. As modular elements of job satisfaction, it has been found that there were personal factors that served to influence satisfaction. In order to determine job satisfaction/dissatisfaction for ASHA professionals, the Job Descriptive Index (JDI) satisfaction score was determined to be the comparator. It indicated that there were areas of dissatisfaction. A multitude of interacting personal variables have been found to be contributory. The coordination of personal needs plays a large part in the level of satisfaction. When the worker is less satisfied, they fulfill significantly fewer human needs. If the worker feels unimportant, job dissatisfaction occurs. However, if their work is accepted as important to the total organization and they are recognized as contributing to the success of the organization, greater satisfaction on the job exists. In other words, part of the job value must be reflected mutually and in levels of service delivery.

The influences and impact are random. Variables such as relationships, gender, job setting, degree of internal satisfaction, societal prestige, and morale can have the same impact on the same job. Features such as positive expectations, less stress, and a sense of freedom will be reduced when the level of fulfillment is high. On the other hand, there may be reduced independence and personal fulfillment. Generally expressed as a personal statement, quality performance and greater satisfaction may be reduced by feeling less in control. The link between job satisfaction/dissatisfaction and problems with speech-language pathologists is often substantiated in the literature. Posters, newsletters, and other published materials can be utilized to increase morale. More professional papers were presented, and numerous contacts were made. This influenced job satisfaction positively. In the area of balanced life which held its place in wellness, self-respect and respect for others were elements in teaching. The lack of respect for both was a concern in the daily working situation, particularly in small country communities. Society also does not respect persons with special needs. As an organization of therapy providers increased, more respect would increase for the individual providers. The more respect a person has, the greater the level of wellness.

CHAPTER 9

Dimensions of Wellness and Their Interconnections

The health dialogue employs a multidimensional approach to understanding and promoting wellness. This approach involves recognizing the interconnectedness of different areas of a person's life and the flow of influence in different directions. At the same time, the health dialogue considers all these areas of life as ego-syntonic: as far as possible, the person should have researched them, understood them, and embraced them. The objective is mental tuning, not moral or aesthetic preaching. The most basic form of wellness is the balance between body, mind, and spirit. Obviously, the so-called spiritual aspects of existence are affected not only by religion and philosophy, but also by our ability to maintain an ethical life and cope with the tasks posed by our personal vocation, with serenity, and without triggering interpersonal irritation, let alone wars.

Health and wellness encompass much more than is commonly understood or accepted, that is, freedom from illness. Health and wellness deal not only with the individual's dealings with personal, cultural, and environmental tasks, but also handle, especially at the political level, the flow of these activities by every person in order to transform life in society into a real health assistance service. Obviously, as a science, medicine deals only with many physical and mental illnesses, but it also needs to provide diagnoses in terms of the individual's and society's performance of human activities. Such performance involves the ability to sidebeam at any particular event in the world and, despite the complexity, to dose the irrational, illogical elements in us, the impossibility of cracking the whole, thus bringing ourselves to the common aeronautical maximum: strip the elements and move forward. Stress, understood as a reaction to change, is just a different therapeutic phenomenon—the unavoidable ratcheting of life.

Understanding the Holistic Nature of Wellness

Health—the one topic that is being spoken about, explained, researched, debated, made fun of, and given utmost priority everywhere. Any number of dialogues or explanations on health are just not enough. On speculating, it could be because many want to remain healthy; to others, it is an industry—a vast, booming business with ample scope; it is life, and its importance is deeply understood. The ways and means to maintain are of utmost importance and a lingering worry to many. The reactions one gets from different walks of life when they see something wrong in your body, surprising as well as agonizing, are testimonies to what is said above. This importance and priority invariably give birth to all forms of dialogues, discussions and knowledge on health, and that is a healthy sign. That opens up doors to scientists both in social and natural sciences to understand and work on the subject. There is no wonder about why people are engaged in research in the area of health and well-being given the amount of importance one attaches to it. These types of research will always have patrons and readers.

We observe that nowadays a huge amount of discussions, dialogues, and research is done in the wellness area initially by business groups, which saw wellness as a service industry; and later, clinical institutions started talking wellness for a different reason. They saw patients who visited them for treatment expressing unhappiness as they were not aware of their health, what caused it, and the path to achieve and remain healthy. The realization started slowly and the wellness industry grew for different reasons. It is important here to ask what wellness is and how different it is from health? An interesting scene happens at the moment these questions get raised. A breed of people from the business, clinical institutions, industry, and institutions all claim that they precisely understood and that health and wellness is all about what they do and what they know. Such a scene is not healthy. Wild and different interpretations are given. Some theorize that health is more to do with bodily functions; a few more argue stating that health is a sign of a few numbers and more related to physical elements; some have gone to the extent to put a dimension to it—health is about physical, mental, social, and spiritual dimensions.

The Synergy Between Different Dimensions
Expanding the Health Dialogue model to include several dimensions of wellness offers a more sophisticated approach to integrative health. The underpinning principle is that different therapeutic approaches relate to different wellness dimensions (essentially, advocating change in one dimension is more relevant to clients or patients who manifest poor health in the same dimension). Fulfilling potential should start with ten fundamental steps, each targeted at the dimension best suited to addressing personal needs. Enhancing problem-solving skills, for example, is a mental health approach,

while advocating regular sleep sufficiency represents a physical health approach.

Practitioners refer to the best experts on other dimensions for help in addressing their personal problems. This does not mean changing a life of addiction or sedentary living before mental and physical health are addressed. The fact that health in a particular dimension may be seriously suboptimal dictates attention to a solution to that very problem. The dialogue between the expert and practitioner shifts focus at that time of life, and the process of change will likely improve health in most, if not all, the other dimensions anyway. Indeed, a focus on just one dimension at a time may reduce the complexity of change and magnify the chance of success.

CHAPTER 10

Barriers to Wellness

Americans worry a lot about our healthcare system. We worry about the cost of care, the quality of care, the waste and incompetence we suspect are common. All this worry leads some of us to suspect that we're somehow missing the point. After all, the reason for the healthcare system's existence, and indeed the only reason for our concern with health, is the desire to ensure individual wellness. So perhaps it's wellness, rather than healthcare, that we ought to be thinking and talking about. If we want to attribute meaning to the healthcare system, we might first require that it be whole. Curative care has been our primary function to date. Holism, the welfare of the whole, is not yet our credo.

We worry about all manner of illnesses, but we put our faith (and our single-minded emphasis) on an industrial-size, gizmo-galore healthcare system, a sick-care system by focus and by nature. We are committed to solving problems of illness rather than achieving goals of wellness. And we are the sorry victims of our rigorous, grossly expensive, over-sophisticated technology. To date, that technology has enabled us to control one or two diseases very well, to treat the sequels of illness with some measure of success, and in a few diseases to prevent or cure. We have also begun to unravel the nature of other illnesses and control some form of healthcare once the link between diagnosis and outcome has been made. Our international business in healing has been increased access of all enfranchised individuals to our cure-oriented productive prowess.

Social Determinants of Health

Health care providers understand, to varying degrees, that lifestyle choices - for example, diet, exercise, and substance use - along with personal life choices - for example, whether to become pregnant and how many children to have - affect a person's health as well as the way any medical intervention is likely to succeed. Often covered in only a small way in health education courses, wellness and the social aspects of health are competing for a more comprehensive approach taken in quality health education materials. In 2003, an Institute of Medicine report formalized this issue. This has helped the conversation with health policymakers who are directed to reduce healthcare costs and health-related costs by keeping people healthy and informed about health.

The 2020 Healthy People information resource describes five key social determinants of health: healthy food and communities, healthy neighborhoods, environmental health, economic community development, and the hotel community affects health and healthcare, addressing inequalities, and does much to increase health and well-being. Some communities are quite innovative. In each community in California where a child is raised, a health score is available to help citizens make informed choices about where to live. Selecting a community with a higher health rating can lead to a child living longer and a better-quality life. Today, many healthcare providers are seeking individuals as patients. Individuals who recognize the long-term benefits of maintaining good health, even when feeling well, and request preventive services or wellness services that might not be covered by health insurance can purchase these services. The cruise line model to prevent diseases, wellness centers operated were a fee-based services on-site medical care and management provide necessary medical care. These services would supplement, not supplant, the primary care received by clients' personal physicians.

Cultural and Societal Factors

Prediction and identification of cultural differences in the manner perceptions of wellness and disease impact a cultural or societal group, and a comprehension of how each individual's cultural or societal group's values affect wellness conclusions form the basis for productive dialogue or mediation. For people from many different cultural, religious, or geographical locations, the term "wellness" has various implications, and acceptance of an individual's or group's perception of healthful living is the beginning point for productive dialogue. For the initial deadline of the Health Dialogue, the starting stage is an appreciation for healthful living and the part of companion animals in healthful living.

In contemporary culture, as witnessed by a rise in Western medication treatments and sporting goods sales, the West is far more involved in Kung Fu and yoga, yet these types of medication treatments are mostly taken out of contexts where these procedures fully express themselves. The effects of the arts such as yoga move far beyond exercise, being fully appreciated only when spiritual acceptability and understanding that this comes. Such examples explain how wellness is particularly refocused at a general level, influenced by the nation of the event, other missions in store, and the command attributes of the minister and the group. In discussions between people of different perspectives, a decent comprehension of societal distinctions is particularly essential for effective mediation. Each side may cause each other to appreciate, maybe value, and possibly take care not to abuse societal and cultural distinctions. From its heritage, the acceptance and regard for individual dignity in the WRC system has been created.

CHAPTER 11

Promoting Wellness: Strategies and Interventions

Promoting wellness is as much about personal choice and action as it is about support from the community and society in general. But this support is rarely given with the same urgency and dedication as when managing sickness and disease. Both the private and public sectors must come together to form an alliance on wellness, or else we are fighting an uphill battle that no one can ever win. Initiatives must be forthright and supplemented with focused funding if they are going to be effective.

The perspective of WHO on the role of the health sector in prevention and promotion can be mentioned with a parallel example of oral health. The strategies and interventions for improving wellness can be personalized and public. It includes educating citizens through the media, training civic leaders and volunteers, developing local networks, providing personal electronic health records, teleconsultation, and finally addressing at the policy level to create a foundation for sustainable wellness. The ultimate goal is to focus on partnerships and results. Such partnership efforts recognize that no single company, seminar, or government can address the challenges of wellness on its own. Efforts as such can be fruitfully developed and revitalized.

Public Health Campaigns and Initiatives

An evaluation of a public health campaign requires attention to the campaign itself – its key components, the overall approach taken, and the messages used – and to any legislation or policies put in place to support or enhance the impacts of the campaign. To evaluate initiatives put in place to address wellbeing or wellness, one may need to look at what supports have been offered within communities or workplaces, and also legislative or policy changes made in Scotland, whether these are ongoing or time-limited, and what the nature of the support offered and the impact has been. The results of the evaluations Health Scotland has carried out suggest a priority for those evaluating public health interventions should be to clarify as fully as possible what was the intention of the intervention.

Public health campaigns – and the initiatives they encourage – are often considered from one of two important perspectives which historically have represented polarized options in medical public health. These perspectives recognize public health activity as focused down either one route or the other. One route involves activity intended to control outbreaks of communicable disease, in response to an acute hazard, and emphasizes what must be done to prevent or control disease or health risk in high-risk groups. The other, more enlightened approach recognizes the importance of wider determinants more generally in the population's health and identifying and addressing health need at an early stage. A good public health campaign might use the language of general determinants in identifying primary, secondary, and tertiary prevention strategies for countering the effects of illness, while at the same time of necessity accepting that more needs to be done to address issues among those particularly at risk of developing disease or illness.

Innovative Technologies for Wellness

As aging-related disparities or complex multimorbidities continue to drive the ever-growing geriatric population who are most vulnerable to chronic diseases, comorbidities lead to increased management and treatment costs. This is driving an enormous demand for medical ICT technologies.

In this chapter, we discussed three key directions of innovative technologies for wellness. The first one is to develop data-driven health intelligence e-systems for monitoring excessive cognitive decline at home. We reviewed the existing projects in this direction, and described some challenges and trends in this field.

The second direction is to develop personal wellness e-systems to model causal effects for early predictors of bodily functions. We provided a data-driven analysis for an innovative personal wellness configuration for wearable IoT devices and a reference model of health state, which can personalize pipelined computation. It should be noted that such consequences brought by a change in an input signal are expected to have different degrees of importance, and the modeling of such a profile using both the domain knowledge and a limited amount of training data for each individual will be quite challenging.

The last direction is to develop comprehensive health management plans by using comprehensive health re-composition technologies, such as caring for skin elderliness, which is often ignored but is very informative.

These 3 promising directions have established a focus on personalized health, to realize the goal in the long run of having the geriatric population engaged in longer and seriously personalized self-management behaviors with their new-generation-expanded nodes in the living environment.

Emerging topics worth researching in the data-driven intelligence for health concise practices include distributing personalized diagnostic machine learning intelligence in the living environment and proposing AI approaches to find subtopic modeling on heterogeneous medical data. In short, the enablers of next-generation data intelligence and smart modeling techniques will likely change the practice of data-driven health in the near future.

With seamless personal health information derived or transferred to personal cloud profiles, these discussed challenges will have to lead to a flourishing ecosystem for a profoundly sophisticated, real-time, predictive early warning system for most dynamics or risky historical individuals.

CHAPTER 12

Measuring Wellness: Tools and Assessments

Interventions focused on improving wellness are best guided by thoughtful assessments of wellness. An assessment can consist of a measurement tool plus an instrument designed to be robust in a very dynamic environment. The latter characteristic is extremely difficult to meet in developing "wellness measures." Initial psychometric properties may be less; however, if a tool is well received by laypersons who can use it effectively, the tool may serve as a good early screen for wellness or its various medical consequences, such as an aspect of learned helplessness, fear of pain, or addictive behaviors. Laypersons seeking to prevent illness and death may benefit by seeking tools designed under more perfectionistic criteria to which wellness researchers are bound.

There are no truly excellent measures of wellness. Many feel a need for an instrument that can quickly and effectively measure this important aspect of our lives. Inexpensive, computer-based data collection has improved this aspect of assessment dramatically. Instead of mailing or telephoning follow-up surveys that only 2/3 of a sample will return, meaning that some samples will have errors that invalidate some data, computer touch screen surveys are available at $4 per hour charge at YMCA's in several different states. Further details may be obtained via the University of Wisconsin Survey Center URL accessible via the University of Wisconsin Office of Health Promotion's Internet home page.

Subjective vs. Objective Measures

Wellness and wellness-related behaviors have been variously defined. Wellness has also been referred to as an intangible or subjective characteristic not easily measured. However, wellness is not unlike other subjective characteristics such as mental attitudes, pain, stress, and satisfaction. Wellness, along with positive attributes such as quality of life and life satisfaction, is emerging as possible goals for health promotion and wellness programs. Certainly, economic and productivity consequences occur when people are not well. Finally, there is a growing interest in assessing how monitoring the fundamental aspects of wellness can help monitor the general health of populations. To date, wellness surveys and analyses of these data have not been performed in the United States or in other countries. Notwithstanding, other countries are clearly ahead of the United States.

There are also differing views on what is meant by wellness among practitioners and researchers. One writer concluded that the failure of health care delivery systems has led laymen as well as professionals to formally explore how one achieves and maintains health. Similarly, some posit that the shift from curative to preventive models of care in this country has been evolving over the past three decades. However, health has been, and remains, the fundamental goal of many clinical analyses. Because some measure of health is the primary goal of most health-producing services and inputs, wellness and quality of life are analyzed largely as subjective outcomes.

Wellness Assessment Scales and Surveys

Wellness assessment tools abound, some concentrating on questionable dimensions or factors. A few robust assessment examples relevant to the fundamental six areas are available. Wellness is definitely multidimensional and the objective is to summarize across the core wellness factors or dimensions such as emotional wellness and sexual wellness. Since the concept not only addresses both feelings and functions, it is important that emotional and sexual intimate normal human behavior does not go untreated just as distress about some somatic disorder is addressed.

Integrating intimate sexual functioning into the arena of emotional wellness is a priority, which is demonstrated by multiple attempts to develop genuine reliable and valid International Index for Sexual Functioning. While designing scales or surveys for standard wellness assessment, the following activities are proposed: 1. Each dimension or factor should be accurately represented. 2. There should be no omission or overlap. 3. The scale should show concurrent criterion validity. 4. The scale should have good internal consistency reliability. 5. It is also advised to examine stability over time although we do realize that wellness is influenced under various circumstances.

CHAPTER 13

The Role of Healthcare Professionals in Wellness

I have learned to appreciate the important property of wellness assets as a result of my experience with many people during the years of my contention with the idea of a culture of optimal health. Most people do try at some level to sustain their state of wellness. They eat, they sleep, they wish to live safe. We now understand that the same beneficial consequences of these ordinary assets and activities can help preserve and enhance their health and that investments in health preservation and enhancement can restore an ill or impaired person to a state of health. I have been asked many times over the years if I expect such a fundamental reform in culture to be implemented in the near future. Of course, I did not at the start and could only hope for the long-term goal to be attained. So, instead of predicting a future outcome, I have developed an answer over the years that includes predictions but provides a present goal that has meaning in and of itself.

One of the old standards for gauging the quality of medical knowledge and care is Florence Nightingale's "What nursing has to do and the wants of the sick it takes to NURSE", the needs of the individual sick person. I have argued for a long while that the next great challenge for medicine is to go beyond the current dominating attitudes and to take responsibility for the nurturing of wellness. Universities should produce professionals who see their mission as nurturing well-being, the nurturing of wellness, and the best investment this country can make today in medicine is making one of the dedicated investments in a support force that will enable health workers to meet the challenge. These are-driven measures to address millions of lives that are cost-effective. With fiber optics, networking, and satellite tracking, patients in their homes are only a heartbeat away. There, they can learn from the advice of professionals. There they can learn you are accountable for your choices and carry out the essential learned wellness responsibility. On this foundation of investments, along with the present Armed Forces Health Professions Scholarship Program, we can build the force to carry on the tradition of Army, Navy, and Public Health Service personnel who have been able to protect us from epidemics of infectious disease. These assets, properly convinced of their importance, can produce a knowledgeable, caring, and responsible system that will do much more to foster the health of the individual and the population wherever such service is outsourced.

Physicians and Nurses

Physicians, also known as doctors, are health professionals who specialize in the practice of medicine. They are responsible for maintaining or restoring human health through diagnosis, treatment, and prevention of disease and injury. In the United States and the Western world, physicians are predominantly educated in the allopathic style of medicine, which has distinct philosophies, practices, and values. Physicians have an extensive background in anatomy, physiology, cell biology, histology, pathology, embryology, immunology, and genetics, and so may practice not only disease-oriented but also wellness-oriented care, while mid-level providers such as nurse practitioners and physician assistants who practice alongside or under a physician's license may be less so. The term physician is used exclusively in the medical field of medicine and should not be confused with a medical practitioner. A medical practitioner is a general term, which commonly encompasses doctors, nurses, and other healthcare professionals, but not medical school graduates or medical office staff.

Nurses, also known as registered nurses, have an extensive background in medical-surgical nursing, maternal-child nursing, psychiatry and mental health nursing, community health nursing, and nursing research. They use all of these skills and practices to assist patients in achieving optimal health and wellness through education, utilization of resources, health promotion, and restoring or maintaining health. Due to their nursing model of care, both preventative and disease-oriented care is often practiced with the help of mid-level practitioners such as Licensed Practical Nurses, Licensed Vocational Nurses, and CNAs (Certified Nursing Assistants). The allopathic model of care is most often practiced by doctors, also known as MD credit physicians, who are specialists in disease rather than wellness, which is most frequently practiced by doctorate-grade nurses who have attended an exclusively nursing school. Training in both models of medicine may increase the overall quality and coverage of a licensed physician, but the doctors' ability to practice wellness may be hindered by their own personal health choices or lifestyles. In contrast, a nurse is an individual who has obtained at least a diploma in nursing (although commonly an Associate's or Bachelor's degree is more educationally favored by medical facilities) and has been licensed to practice after passing a national board. Upon graduation from a nursing program, some seasoned nurses informally mentor or precept new nurses about ethical standards and patient care practices. They help such novice nurses process information and make decisions by explaining choices made and resolving any problems that may arise, following a particular set of guidelines known as written standards of operations.

Mental Health Practitioners

Mental health practitioners, whether minister, psychiatrist, or psychologist, need to be attuned to the issues of safety, security, and death that are so poignant to the processes of health dialogues. Additionally, they need to put aside their clinging to models and theories and allow reality to guide their empathic behavior. The cultivation of mastery over their natural roles is an important task, for their own effectiveness and their avoidance of unhealthy transference and counter-transference roles. Additionally, they need models of human nature that view citizenship behavior as basic to the human psyche, for normal behavior transcends the limitations of one's natural roles. The assertion of the human being is regarded as normal behavior, whereas people who accept imposed limits to the expression of themselves are regarded as disturbed, whether or not they behave in ways dictated by professional models derived from philosophical or religious belief structures.

As a matter of clarification, a minister can be viewed as a community leader who promotes the quality of life of the parish congregation, or as a spiritual teacher who administers to the inner self of the parishioner. A minister may take on hybrid community leader/spiritual teacher responsibilities, and may shift roles given the time and place. In many small Protestant churches, the ministers take on the shopkeeper's duties also. These dual roles define the extraordinary adaptability and affective modeling skills of ministers. As a community leader, he would counsel with parishioners on issues relating to their family and workplace roles. Issues which involve emotional distress are the jurisdiction of a spiritual teacher who performs, in large part, the comforting function and not the problem-solving skills of a leader. In the scholarly/mentor role, the minister may function in the educational process, and through sermons, scripts, lectures, and study classes act as counselor and problem-solver. Of the three helping roles, being a spiritual facilitator is by far the most demanding role and is least capable of being formally defined. The advanced technologies used by the federal government as well as psychoanalysis are but poor replacements for this extraordinary human talent. Except for help in the healing of extremely severe illness models of practitioners, the leader and teacher and community builders would meet the emotional coincubines and the congregants of the spiritual realms. Ministers are the outgrowth of ancient social tradition. The ability to perform essential emotional roles is the key to a successful career as a social leader, teacher, and community builder. According to the United States Department of Labor, one-third of the human service workers today are ministerial personnel.

CHAPTER 14

Wellness in Different Population Groups

As presented in other parts of this book, the concept of wellness can extend to groups and populations. Progress and development are key components in fostering mental and emotional health. Also, promoting an encouraging environment for wellness to blossom, as well as ensuring that one is equipped with the necessary coping mechanisms as one changes in life, are of great importance. At this global level, it is equally important to negotiate civil and authoritative structures and to influence the political, social, cultural, economic, technological, and environmental aspects of our civilization that affect our lives.

Given the great diversity of local and cultural needs, the descriptions of wellness for the different population groups are only illustrative. Many different population groups are to be found within countries, and these discuss some of those who organize gatherings to help establish wellness concepts and practice as needed. The examples selected vary from national leadership to the welfare and wellness of families and from aging to skilled and productive cultures of people. These groups have very different needs in terms of wellness, but at the same time, they have to work together, sometimes in organizations with people involved in more than one of these activities. Only through strong, healthy, and relevant organizations can society advance with responsive leadership to help guide change, reducing uncertainty and adopting relevant solutions to global problems while maintaining people and their cultures and civilizations.

Children and Adolescents

The mental and physical health of children is often linked with the health of family members. A family-oriented approach can help to develop and implement more effective health-promotion programs for children. Typical programs aimed at helping children address health risks often show only modest benefits. By focusing on the family, the potential for improving child health increases. Changes in eating, exercise, and health habits in overweight adolescents are often better when the entire family, including siblings, becomes involved. The family-oriented approach pairs relevant information with the kind of social support systems that have been shown to produce positive behavior change.

Adolescents stand on the brink of adulthood. They experience both opportunity and vulnerability as they explore different aspects of their lives. Since what they learn by experience forms their future health attitudes and behaviors, the priority for adolescents is to balance risk with independence, and offer access to good and timely information that encourages responsible behavior for them. Adolescents also need to feel good about themselves and respect others. See also Chapter 2, Our Children and Families; Chapter 5, Assessing and Choosing Health Care Services; Chapter 11, Disease-and Health-Risk-Focused Programs; Chapter 13, Empowering Teenagers.

Elderly Population

Now let us review these special needs for the elderly population. Just as anticipated, the major concern with respect to seniors is that of death. Unlike the population at large that takes a bad disease or other forms of accidental death as the first priority, seniors seem more concerned with dying because they feel they have lived long enough, or now have a limited quality of life. They are, however, concerned at which state of health death occurs. For most, it is during their sleep. This highly contrasts with the general population that would like to prevent dying during sleep, for fear of dying. Another interesting point with respect to seniors is that most perceive our present world as 'ugly', environmentally speaking. They feel their past world was much simpler and return often to complain that we are depleting our natural resources irrationally. Their vision of wellness includes quality of life options right up to the very end of their lives.

This concern with respect to health and wellness issues representing true quality of life is not justional, however. Most seniors attend their appointments faithfully, continually expressing their concerns with respect to today's medical treatments. The fact that chronic degenerative diseases of old age are far from being resolved and demand long-term commitments on a daily basis make those wellness strategies of prime importance, seeing them quite clearly as contributors to an improvement of their quality of life. Their inquiry on the matter is constant. The matter of being surrounded by their family and community in general, representing only five percent of the research population, was highlighted as quality enhancements to their wellness strategies, being presented under the interface of a pluricentric wellness program, representing a life continuum. On the negative side, not being aware of existing wellness strategies for the better or a particular health problem not being handled satisfactorily top off the negative end of the scale.

Minority and Marginalized Communities

The following types of health disparities have been documented through a range of research methods and they represent a few of the multiple facets of minority and multicultural experiences that introduce profound health challenges into wellness and disease prevention: environmental control of health. The health disparities found between different racial, ethnic, and other vulnerable populations may reflect the direct health-affecting impacts from adverse environments. Poor environmental quality appears to be an important but often overlooked determinant of increased chronic illness rates in poor and marginalized populations, particularly related to respiratory health and the increased prevalence and severity of asthma-related illnesses. The impact of environmental toxins and pollution appears to be a major cause of women's health disparities, maternal and infant mortality, low birth weight, average deficiencies, and disparities in development, cognitive inhibitory, and neurobehavioral function.

"Have yours" is the response from the recognized cultures and minorities; "their programs certainly don't seem to be working for me". Though necessary for equity, it is not only the easier access to resources and programs that are required to address problems but usually better programming. In programs that strive for beneficial behavior change regardless of a person's approach to life, culture does not matter. Successful programs do not need to be political in nature, nor do programs need to create their own materials simply because standard cultural references are not used, but they do need to be culturally sensitive and respectful. Successful programs require the development of a belief in and appreciation for knowledge programs and a feeling of genuine concern for the safety, health, and welfare of persons from all walks of life in every community within a society. Personalization of programs is at the heart of addressing life cycles, cultures, characteristics, health risks, concerns, and experiences in a meaningful manner.

CHAPTER 15

Wellness in the Workplace

Many employers are recognizing the need for workplace wellness programs, which strive to help employees lead healthier lifestyles and maintain positive health outcomes. Not only does a good corporate wellness program have a positive impact on employee health, but other advantages can also result, including improved productivity and job satisfaction levels. However, success only comes from individuals who are motivated to live moderate, balanced lives. It is imperative that corporate wellness programs don't stifle this internal motivation within people. Even though these types of programs are getting more and more popular, organizations need to give careful consideration before implementing their own wellness programs. Not every company is poised to capitalize on implementing a corporate wellness program, although the potential paybacks of this type of action could be high.

Research on the effectiveness of corporate wellness programs has been mixed. Although there are many proponents of corporate wellness programs, it will take careful planning and strategic implementation for something of this nature to work. Care messages, suggesting free alternatives for the purpose of managing health, "Free" puts the individual in control; it's a liberating feeling. Program managers, initially scared of letting go, are realizing that they need their health consumers more than health consumers need them, at least to reach initial tipping that sets the wheel into motion for a more responsive, cost-effective health care system. With a real need to put wellness in hybrid consumer hands, wellness at the workplace faces the dichotomous challenge of carelessness (as benefits of vertical care have tightened up) and organizational care. The bottom line to the organization is productivity and health care cost containment. The employee/social-cared citizen is ultimately responsible for personal health care choices.

Corporate Wellness Programs

The advent of the industrial age began to wrestle power away from the traditional economic empires of the landed gentry, the church, and royalty. The Industrial and Technological Age has lost its initial habits of oppression as consensus and economic democratization become frequent companions and the extremes at either end of the fairness spectrum begin to balance. There are unfortunately flaws and growing pains attendant with growing older and stronger. An unerring mastery of matter has also been recognized for what it is - powerful; knowledge can in the wrong hands become manipulation and unbridled materialism can become sick. Consequently, the true drivers of economic health, the people, require nurturing and guidance toward the concept of wellness.

It is both impractical and absurd to expect people to function consistently or for any length of time efficiently and responsibly if their minds are on their health or even the health of their families. It is simply far more economical to apologize for poor health than to try to do something constructive about the basic cause - neglect of health. Consequently, the trend has been toward the development of the Total Compensation approach to employee benefits. The individual is viewed as part of a total unit comprised of financing, health care, protection, and retirement programs both voluntary and federally supported. Each aspect of the Total Compensation Plan supports the other and represents a vital part of the employee's personal welfare and welfare of his family. To be truly effective the employee must understand and participate in using the plan, which requires interest and a high degree of confidence in the employer's efforts. Providing proper service should be a goal rather than a necessity. If employer service is not available the employee is not fully serviced and the purpose of the program is diminished if not destroyed.

Ergonomics and Workplace Design

Health and wellness are fundamental considerations in the Fairfax County wellness program. The working environment is a key component in the health and wellness of staff. In a portion of data located in Appendix D, a few specific considerations are addressed, but the list is not exhaustive. These cover a wide range of areas from ergonomic considerations, HVAC systems, and audio, visual, interactive, and written related areas. A few sources also provide some step-checklists that may be beneficial in the new building or remodeling stages for management groups to consider in the wellness capacity assessments that are part of working to meet the objectives and strategies of the Health and Wellness Plan.

Fairfax County's employee population is subject to the same principles. When an employee is injured on the job, when an employee works with pain because their work station does not allow them to have an appropriate anthropometric neutral zone, when an employee contracts a communicable illness due to the work environment, or when an employee is just plain uncomfortable, they suffer a great deal, and their ability to service the public is also compromised. The answer may be a physical wellness space or other types of ergonomic responses that facilitate keeping one at work.

CHAPTER 16

Global Perspectives on Wellness

These seven global views represent a range of viewpoints on wellness from those currently representing a particular sector, either independent or as a constituent group of society. Each global view is positioned in the larger context of current societal evolution, and subsequently their contribution is recognized in the journey to make wellness an achievable reality. Essentially, wellness is introduced without pre-definitions of its essence, such as 'quality of life' or health or fitness, since predefined essence inhibits creativity and standpoint. Over time, constituent individual wellness measurable variables have become known and are relatively easy to establish at individual, community, and macro levels of society.

The five dimensions of wellness - structural, mental, physical, emotional, and spiritual - often determine the behavior within specific sectors. Hence, when considering the whole spectrum of wellness, looking at specific sectors also contributes to a global view. The global views are coordinated from the perspective that in today's society, many sectors function in somewhat staid, time-lagged, or silo mode as each seeks situational performance improvement, while other sectors are embarking on an evolutionary wellness journey that is achieved through cultural/environmental interaction. When the cultural/environmental interaction of sector endeavors is experienced by society, then the concept of society sharing and learning from the wellness journey expands the achievement horizon.

Cross-Cultural Variations in Wellness Practices

The goal of exploring the role of culture in wellness practices so far has been a limited one: to determine if variations do indeed exist, and if so, to describe them roughly and in what areas. This first exploration has been very useful, however. It serves in a sense as a feasibility study suggesting that culture does indeed play a major role. Further, from the level one analysis comes much of the power behind cultural techniques for wellness. The sizable differences resulted in solutions from quite different cultures that emphasize the differences. Only after looking at these cultural perspectives does the full power of the work really become clear. Loads of hints about these can be seen by noticing the differences. It seems clear that a level 2 examination, exploring the specific mechanisms by which these differences are created and can be utilized, would confirm this intuition and be useful in the development of better wellness programs.

As expected from these activities, it did appear that different cultures isolated distinct levels of feeling and that the specific ways in which these levels were distinguished differed by culture. This cross-cultural variation was not at the levels of the Maxwell multiple intelligences. Several, and in several cases many, of the different cultures continued to agree. That is, the isolation of multiple levels became the next source of wellness programs tried. And after the different wellness solutions were isolated, it was these different, multiple level demands that provided the clues to developing appropriate wellness programs. In some cases, some of the levels, although distinguished, were nonetheless grouped. Individuals from these cultures gave similar wellness responses, and what appeared at first to be two or more wellness levels really appeared to be just one.

International Health Policies and Wellness

The last two decades have seen an increased involvement on the part of governments in the management of their own health systems. There are many reasons for this. Given the assumption that people have an inalienable right to life, many governments have, for a variety of reasons, accepted as part of their responsibilities the task of guaranteeing their citizens access to basic levels of health care. Also, modern definitions of health incorporate social and psychological values alongside organic wellbeing, which obliges health professionals to help establish the necessary conditions. The nonexistence or weakness of health infrastructures in many developing countries has meant that, in the absence of national systems for the provision of services, private networks are systematically described as being both the major existing providers and the legitimate heirs to be financed by public policy.

Although policy creation in health is an increasingly internationalized subject, three specifics of the major transformations now being experienced need to be emphasized. First, unlike the case for economic developments set out in many other works, the intrusive role of states in the health system during and after the 1939-1945 war is still very present in policy-making for many countries, which means that we shall have to analyze it specifically. Second, the differences between health care in either developed or less favored countries are each as important, numerous, and transversal. Finally, as with the other public policies, the unforeseen consequences of global epidemiological pressures need to be mentioned.

CHAPTER 17

Ethical Considerations in Wellness Promotion

In the health promotion literature, it is assumed that everyone should be given the opportunity to achieve an appropriate level of general well-being. A common fuel for the promotion of health and wellness is the need to reduce healthcare expenditure, which means that major employers are also involved in health promotion.

The purpose of this chapter is to demonstrate that it might be possible to increase the level of wellness by promoting choice itself. In other words, as an alternative to a political, educational, and behavioral approach to health promotion, we may need to consider the actual effects of the thought that constructs well-being. The literature in Heidegger (1962), Cassirer (2002), and Wittgenstein (2003) suggests an integration of therapy and wellness, and the promotion of this integrated approach may be the fuel that leads to an increase in the overall spiritual health and wellness of a population.

Reality and Wellness The debate on the relationship between human beings and their sexual orientation is made complex by the fact that sexual identity is the combination of not only our physical sex but also our physical experience with our body, and our affection, attachment, and sexual orientation. Often, the sense of disagreement between the body and the individual crosses the strictly physical position of the body and may originate what some philosophers have called the state of disembodiment. First of all, there is the philosophical idea that often creates distress in the individual coming from the comparison between one's physical image and that which the ideal model of beauty, proposed and imposed by culture, establishes.

Informed Consent and Privacy

Privacy is certainly one of the predominant issues of concern when dealing with any database and the information contained therein. The proprietary rights to those data are likely to be of no small concern, and there are significant issues with regard to the quality of demographic and other pertinent non-health data. Organizations providing access to information systems, researchers seeking to use that information, and individuals having their information contained in the database all have significant concerns that relate to privacy. It is clear that the essential legitimacy of most uses of these data can be made to depend upon sensitivity to these real concerns about the confidentiality of what otherwise seem to be routine health care surveillance tools.

In our view, the basic construct providing legitimacy to these database systems is the agreement of the citizens of any political jurisdiction to consent to and pay on an ongoing basis for the third-party utilization of these tools as an ongoing surveillance system. This exchange forms the foundation of the "implied consent/limited permission" model for the use of medical record-based "administrative" data for the important functions of quality assessment and cost-efficiency analysis. The democratic process creates an open forum for an ongoing dialogue on such issues and defines a space wherein the intersubjective patterns and meanings that address these issues are continuously evolving. Given our political and economic system, this is a likely configuration of interests and outcomes.

Avoiding Harm and Exploitation

Certainly, in realist metatheoretical terms, this underlying reference to our capacity to exist without manipulating others' distress provides a normative consideration informing our ontological existence. It is a key issue that has relevance to our reflexive sustaining of the social fabric upon which a "holistic" state of wellness can exist. When referring to positive individual states of "well-being" (as distinct from the collective "wellness" of society), self-fulfillment or eudemonia refers to an abstract, ideal state of humanity characterized by dynamic activity, self-realization, autonomy, self-sufficiency, and freedom. These are characteristic factors that signal being on "top of the world", in good psychic health, meaning there is no impediment to complete individual self-determination, an ideal state of individual wellness, with "no barriers to the achievement of one's highest ambitions".

CHAPTER 18

Future Directions in Wellness Research and Practic

Knowing that a more comprehensive knowledge of wellness as a human phenomenon should inform policy creation and the development and interpretation of educational systems at all ages, Heritage's conclusion to his exploration of the fundamental aspects of human wellness, under the intriguing title "Believing Impossible Things Before Breakfast" - with reference to the character of Lewis Carroll's Through the Looking-Glass - addressed the need for an expanded recognition and conceptual understanding of the personal enterprise dimensions of the wellness construct that can allow a more complete comprehension of their hyperdimensional qualities and catalytic effects in human lives. He suggested several possible alternative levels of inquiry that can be explored in order to broaden and deepen the phenomenological roots of wellness and make them even more extraordinary - namely by (a) taking into account the range and character of the presuppositions we use in framing the construct of wellness, (b) by considering evidence about the activity of effect as an iterative quality that inhales all fields of evidence and practice.

The emphasis is clearly on clarifying thoughts and typologies that are, while generalizable, extremely variable, and by contributing towards the establishment of some operational principles for future research in creating and interpreting constructs known under the common heading of "wellness", in the particular/fiddler/latticewise/fuzzy/complex/collapsing/diverse/elusive landscape of human experience. These are major research challenges that have the potential to effect significant contributions for our understanding of human behavior in all healthcare-related research and application domains. Particularly, he called for new longitudinal or within-subjects - not intermodules designs that would investigate particular dimensions and aspects of wellness to operationalize the holistic nature of the construct, to investigate the ebb flow major/minor instability, variability, fatigue, decay, dis/equilibrium, culminating processes, and (some) non-normative behavior.

Emerging Trends and Innovations

The consumer's demand for health and wellness services has continued to gain strength over the past two decades. This change in demand has, in turn, altered the ways in which health care organizations and other providers define, measure, provide, and communicate wellness. As health care organizations confront increasing competition from both traditional corporate providers and new non-traditional providers for their constituents in existing and new markets, many are developing special services and products, including health and wellness fairs, wellness resource centers, nutrition classes, and information lines. Such endeavors are to meet this new challenge by integrating wellness throughout their patient care and preventative educational programs.

Increasingly, health care organizations are incorporating health promotion and wellness into their fundamental missions as well.

They are doing so, in part, through affiliation with health care organizations that have proven experience in providing health and wellness services; and they are supporting, in increasing numbers, the creation of health and wellness referral centers. In addition, more health boards are reflecting wellness interests through the establishment of standing wellness subcommittees. In short, they are responding to the growing needs, interests, and activities of today's consumer.

Interdisciplinary Approaches to Wellness

Physicians often criticize psychiatry for being longitudinal instead of dealing with the central problems of the here and now. Psychiatry is perceived as dealing with regressive behavior, inconsistencies of perception, disturbances of the here and now. To what extent can an instructor in interpersonal skills respond favorably to these sorts of questions - or should he challenge them? That is, either challenge the questioner as a blocking symptom or state that cognition and affect and behavior and perception are integral units, interrelated with each other. There is universal consensus that the best treatment is one that efficiently handles the present. Since man has conscious awareness, he can be described as being present-centered. None of our treatments are unmodified and therefore can be termed depth therapies. Yet most of the teaching in cost-effective health care is symptom-focused. These patients come for health care because they have specific concerns: they are responding to anxiety about their health. They place an international demand on consultant-liaison services.

Most in-office, off-the-street health problems are transient. Gee - thanks, I feel so much better, Doc; confounding interpretations are ordered. We commonly ask a patient about his relief from the Intracellular Membrane Complex Marker Diagnostic Test that indicates that we care more about him and the patient is convinced we don't care at all, except by handling him, but our behavior is systematic and intentional. The closed office practice is, then, largely activated by and scheduled around transient health problems. Such problems are familiar to the practitioner - and they are consoling and satisfying for the recipient. Let's examine briefly some of the practical and intuitive problems implicit in that art and science. Medical school officers, practice-direction counselors, house officers, psychiatry residents, and practice-minded sociology students - particularly if they are restricted to half-hour, once-a-week meetings for six months or a year, or weeks that change their patients from one hour to another and by rotation change their hours between 9 a.m. and 3:00 p.m., Monday through orifices in the bodies of various people, 5_6 - are prone to observational myopia and undertaking philosophically modeled health gain approaches.

CHAPTER 19

Conclusion: Key Takeaways and Implications for Hea

In this chapter and throughout this book, we have considered the increasing nexus between the fields of health promotion/health communication and wellness and have explored how wellness is incorporated into The Health Dialogue. The overall objective of this book and particularly this chapter is to present the fundamental aspects of wellness and consider how the applicability of these aspects to the online evidence-based health and wellness program, The Health Dialogue, may be related to health.

To conclude this chapter, the fundamental aspects of wellness reviewed in this chapter are highly comprehensive. These aspects relate to almost all areas of living and are relevant to people of all ages. The fundamental aspects of wellness reviewed in this chapter are presented in Table 19.1. The importance of wellness and how wellness ties in with health communication and health promotion has been presented. This has highlighted the importance of the consideration of wellness and its relevant aspects in technology-based programs. Support has been given for the applicability of programs for the older population. The rationale for considering wellness in the review of The Health Dialogue has been provided based on the growth in research advocating the consideration of this important human construct.